Essential

FAST

FEAST REPEAT

Cookbook

Celebrate Flavorful Weight Loss with Quick and Easy Recipes for Delicious Feasts, Speedy Culinary Creations, and Everyday Feast Favorites

MARIYAM MOHL

Copyright © 2023 by Mariyam Mohl

TABLE OF CONTENT

INTRODUCTION

We frequently find ourselves at a crossroads in a society where time is a valuable resource and leading a healthful lifestyle is more vital than ever. When our days are filled with a flurry of fast-paced activities and responsibilities, it might feel impossible to maintain a balanced diet and lose those excess pounds.

This is where the "Essential Fast Feast Repeat Cookbook" comes in—it serves as a reliable guide for long-term weight loss and improved health in addition to being a delightful recipe book. With this cookbook's special combination of speed and nutrition, you can indulge in your favorite flavors without compromising the value of your day's most important moments.

The word "Fast" in our title refers to an effective weight reduction strategy rather than merely rapid preparation. You'll learn that you don't need to follow fad diets or spend a lot of time in the kitchen to reach your health and fitness objectives. We've carefully selected meals that will help you on your weight reduction journey in addition to being handy.

The word "feast" in our title refers to the wide range of tastes and variations our cookbook provides. It doesn't have to be boring or monotonous to eat for weight reduction. Enjoy an abundance of delicious cuisine that satisfy your palate and replenish your body. You'll see from our dishes that eating healthily doesn't have to mean restriction.

The secret to long-term success is "Repeat". We think that durability and consistency have great power. With the help of our cookbook, you can make well-informed decisions for your health that you can stick with and eventually incorporate into your daily routine. This is a route to long-term transformation, not a band-aid solution.

Come along for the ride as we explore the world of quick, tasty, and diet-friendly dishes. With the help of the "Essential Fast Feast Repeat Cookbook," you may adopt a better lifestyle without compromising your valuable time. Together, we will embark on your weight reduction journey, one delectable meal at a time.

Pasta Primavera Recipe

Ingredients:

For the Pasta:

- 8 oz (225g) of your favorite pasta (e.g., spaghetti, fettuccine, or penne)
- Salt, for boiling water

For the Primavera Sauce:

- 2 tablespoons olive oil
- 2 cloves garlic, minced
- 1 small red onion, thinly sliced
- 1 bell pepper, thinly sliced (use a mix of colors for added visual appeal)
- 1 small zucchini, thinly sliced
- 1 cup cherry tomatoes, halved
- 1 cup broccoli florets
- 1/2 cup snap peas or green beans, trimmed
- 1/4 cup fresh basil leaves, torn
- Salt and black pepper, to taste
- Grated Parmesan cheese, for garnish (optional)

Instructions:

1. Boil the Pasta:
- Cook the pasta as directed on the box until it's al dente. Drain and put aside.
- Bring a large pot of salted water to a boil.
2. Prepare the Primavera Sauce:
- Heat the olive oil in a big pan over medium heat.

- ➢ Add the minced garlic and cook, stirring, until fragrant, approximately 30 seconds.
- ➢ Include the bell pepper and red onion slices. Cook for two to three minutes, or until they begin to get tender.

Add Vegetables:

- Fill the skillet with the zucchini, cherry tomatoes, broccoli florets, and snap peas (or green beans).
- Sauté the veggies for five to seven minutes, or until they are crisp-tender. Put some salt and black pepper over it.

Combine Pasta and Sauce:

- Toss everything to incorporate, then add the cooked pasta and the sautéed veggies to the pan.

Finish and Serve:

- Turn off the heat and add the freshly torn basil leaves to the skillet.
- If necessary, taste and add additional salt and black pepper to the seasoning.
- If preferred, top the heated Pasta Primavera with grated Parmesan cheese.

Benefits:

- Packed with nutrients: Pasta primavera has an abundance of different veggies that provide vital vitamins, minerals, and fiber.

- Low in saturated fat: This recipe is healthier since it utilizes olive oil rather than heavy cream or butter.
- Customizable: You may change the veggies used according to your tastes or what's in season.

Applications:

- Pasta primavera is a flexible recipe that may be eaten as a main course by vegetarians on its own. Tofu, shrimp, or even grilled chicken can be added for additional protein.
- It is a great side dish for special occasions or to serve at potlucks and family feasts.

Chicken Stir-Fry Recipe

Ingredients:

For the Stir-Fry Sauce:

- 3 tablespoons soy sauce
- 2 tablespoons oyster sauce
- 1 tablespoon hoisin sauce
- 1 tablespoon rice vinegar
- 1 tablespoon honey or brown sugar
- 1 teaspoon cornstarch

For the Stir-Fry:

- 2 boneless, skinless chicken breasts, thinly sliced
- 2 tablespoons vegetable oil
- 1 red bell pepper, thinly sliced
- 1 yellow bell pepper, thinly sliced
- 1 cup broccoli florets
- 1 carrot, thinly sliced
- 1 cup snap peas, trimmed
- 3 cloves garlic, minced
- 1-inch piece of fresh ginger, minced
- Cooked rice or noodles for serving
- Sesame seeds and chopped green onions for garnish (optional)

Instructions:

Prepare the Stir-Fry Sauce:

- Combine the soy sauce, hoisin sauce, oyster sauce, rice vinegar, honey (or brown sugar), and cornstarch in a small basin. Reserve the sauce.

Cook the Chicken:

- In a big skillet or wok, heat up 1 tablespoon of vegetable oil over medium-high heat.
- When the chicken is no longer pink in the center, add the sliced chicken to the skillet and cook for about 4–5 minutes. After removing it from the pan, set the chicken aside.

Stir-Fry the Vegetables:

- Add the final tablespoon of vegetable oil to the same skillet.
- Stir-fry the ginger and garlic for 30 seconds or until aromatic.
- Include the snap peas, broccoli, carrot, and cut red and yellow bell peppers. Stir-fry the veggies for 3–4 minutes, or until they are crisp-tender.

Combine and Finish:

- Add the cooked chicken and the sautéed veggies back to the skillet.
- Drizzle the chicken and veggies with the stir-fried sauce.
- Combine all the ingredients and simmer for a further two to three minutes, so the sauce can coat and thicken the food.

Serve:

- Plate the hot chicken stir-fry over noodles or cooked rice.
- If preferred, garnish with chopped green onions and sesame seeds.

Benefits:

- High in Protein: Packed with protein, this stir-fried chicken dish is a filling and healthy meal.
- Loaded with Vegetables: An array of vibrant vegetables contributes vital vitamins and minerals.
- Customizable: You can modify the vegetables and sauce to your preferred taste.

Applications:

- Serve chicken stir-fried with a variety of rice dishes (white, brown, or cauliflower rice) or noodles for a quick and healthful meal.
- It's also a great way to use up leftover vegetables from your fridge. You can even make it vegetarian by replacing the chicken with tofu or tempeh.

Taco Salad Recipe

Ingredients:

For the Taco Seasoning:

- 1 tablespoon chili powder
- 1 teaspoon ground cumin
- 1/2 teaspoon paprika
- 1/2 teaspoon garlic powder
- 1/2 teaspoon onion powder
- 1/4 teaspoon crushed red pepper flakes (adjust to taste)
- 1/4 teaspoon dried oregano
- Salt and black pepper to taste

For the Salad:

- 1 lb (450g) ground beef or turkey
- 1 can (15 oz) black beans, drained and rinsed
- 1 cup corn kernels (fresh, frozen, or canned)
- 1 cup cherry tomatoes, halved
- 1 cup shredded cheddar or Mexican blend cheese
- 1/2 cup sliced black olives
- 1/2 cup diced red onion
- 1/4 cup chopped fresh cilantro
- 1/4 cup sour cream
- 1/4 cup salsa
- Tortilla chips or strips for garnish
- Lime wedges for serving (optional)

Instructions:

Prepare the Taco Seasoning:

- Combine the chili powder, cumin, paprika, onion powder, garlic powder, dried oregano, red pepper flakes, salt, and black pepper in a small bowl. Put away the taco seasoning.

Cook the Meat:

- Brown and fully cook the ground beef or turkey in a large pan over medium-high heat.
- After the meat has cooked, drain any extra fat and mix in the taco spice. To thoroughly coat the meat with the spice, stir. After lowering the heat to low, simmer it for a short while.

Assemble the Salad:

- Arrange the items in the following order in a large salad bowl:
- Lay a bed of tortilla strips or chips first.

Incorporate the spiced pork.

- Top with black beans, red onion, cilantro, corn, cherry tomatoes, cheese, and black olives.
- Pour salsa and sour cream over the salad.
- Present the taco salad with extra tortilla strips or chips on top.
- You may perhaps provide lime wedges for the salad to be dressed with.

Benefits:

- Protein: The ground beef contains protein, which is necessary for the development and maintenance of muscles.

- Nutrients and Fiber: The salad's black beans and veggies provide vitamins, minerals, and fiber.
- Customizable: You may make it as healthy or decadent as you'd like by changing the toppings and ingredients to fit your tastes.

Applications:

- Taco salad is a great lunch or supper option as it is a whole meal in and of itself.
- It makes a tasty and enjoyable meal to serve at get-togethers, potlucks, and parties.
- It's a great way to use up components from leftover tacos.

Veggie Quesadillas Recipe

Ingredients:

For the Veggie Filling:

- 1 bell pepper, thinly sliced (use a mix of colors for variety)
- 1 red onion, thinly sliced
- 1 cup sliced mushrooms
- 1 cup baby spinach leaves
- 1 cup shredded cheddar or Monterey Jack cheese
- 1 tablespoon olive oil
- Salt and black pepper, to taste

For the Quesadillas:

- 4 large flour tortillas
- 2 tablespoons butter (for cooking)
- Salsa, sour cream, or guacamole for serving (optional)

Instructions:

Prepare the Veggie Filling:

- Heat the olive oil in a big pan over medium heat.
- Include the red onion, mushrooms, and bell pepper slices in the skillet. Vegetables should be sautéed for 5 to 7 minutes, or until they are soft and slightly browned. Put some salt and black pepper over it.
- Cook the baby spinach in the pan for a further one to two minutes, or until it has wilted. Take the skillet off of the burner.

Assemble the Quesadillas:

- Melt half of the butter in a big pan or griddle over medium heat.
- Place one flat tortilla in the griddle and top with 1/4 of the cheese that has been shredded.
- Spoon some of the vegetable filling that has been sautéed over the cheese.
- Place a second tortilla on top.
- Cook for two to three minutes on each side, or until the cheese has melted and the tortilla is golden brown. Using a spatula, press down to ensure the quesadilla stays together.
- Continue the procedure with the remaining tortillas, cheese, and vegetable filling.

Serve:
- Take out of the griddle and allow the quesadillas to cool for a minute before slicing into wedges.
- If preferred, serve hot with guacamole, sour cream, or salsa on the side.

Benefits:
- Vegetarian: A tasty and wholesome alternative to vegetarian meals are veggie quesadillas.
- Rich in Fiber and Nutrients: A range of vitamins, minerals, and fiber are provided by the combination of bright veggies.

- Customizable: You may customize the quesadillas to your liking by adding more veggies or seasonings.

Applications:

- Especially for those on a vegetarian or meatless diet, veggie quesadillas can be presented as a delicious lunch or supper option.
- They make a terrific appetizer, snack, or light meal.
- Perfect for simple, quick weeknight dinners that you can alter the ingredients to fit whatever you have on hand.

Veggie Quesadillas Recipe

Ingredients:

For the Veggie Filling:

- 1 red bell pepper, thinly sliced
- 1 green bell pepper, thinly sliced
- 1 red onion, thinly sliced
- 1 zucchini, thinly sliced
- 1 cup sliced mushrooms
- 2 cups baby spinach leaves
- 2 cloves garlic, minced
- 2 tablespoons olive oil
- Salt and black pepper, to taste

For the Quesadillas:

- 4 large flour tortillas
- 2 cups shredded cheese (cheddar, Monterey Jack, or your choice)
- Cooking spray or extra olive oil for cooking

For Serving (optional):

- Salsa
- Sour cream
- Guacamole

Instructions:

Prepare the Veggie Filling:

- Heat the olive oil in a big pan over medium heat.
- Fill the skillet with the sliced bell peppers, red onion, zucchini, and mushrooms. Vegetables should be sautéed for 5 to 7 minutes, or until they are soft and slightly

browned. Put some salt and black pepper over it.

- Include the chopped garlic and cook for an additional 30 seconds, or until aromatic.
- Cook the baby spinach in the pan for a further one to two minutes, or until it has wilted. Take the skillet off of the burner.

Assemble the Quesadillas:

- Heat up a sizable pan or griddle over medium heat and coat it with a little amount of olive oil or cooking spray.
- Place one flat tortilla in the griddle and top with 25% of the cheese that has been shredded.
- Transfer some of the sautéed vegetable filling to the cheese.
- Place a second tortilla on top.
- Cook for two to three minutes on each side, or until the cheese has melted and the tortilla is golden brown. Using a spatula, press down to ensure the quesadilla stays together.
- Continue with the remaining tortillas, cheese, and vegetable filling.

Serve:

- Take out of the griddle and allow the quesadillas to cool for a minute before slicing into wedges.
- If preferred, serve hot with guacamole, salsa, or sour cream on the side.

Benefits:

- Vegetarian: A tasty and wholesome alternative to vegetarian meals are veggie quesadillas.
- Rich in Fiber and Nutrients: A range of vitamins, minerals, and fiber are provided by the combination of bright veggies.
- Customizable: You may customize the quesadillas to your liking by adding more veggies or seasonings.

Applications:

- Especially for those on a vegetarian or meatless diet, veggie quesadillas can be presented as a delicious lunch or supper option.
- They make a terrific appetizer, snack, or light meal.
- Perfect for simple, quick weeknight dinners that you can alter the ingredients to fit whatever you have on hand.

Caprese Salad Recipe

Ingredients:

- 4 ripe tomatoes, preferably vine-ripened or heirloom
- 8 ounces (about 2 cups) fresh mozzarella cheese, sliced
- 1 bunch fresh basil leaves
- Extra-virgin olive oil
- Balsamic glaze (optional)
- Salt and freshly ground black pepper, to taste

Instructions:

1. Prepare the Ingredients:

- Rinse the tomatoes and cut them into rounds that are 1/4 inch thick.
- Cut the fresh mozzarella cheese into rounds that are 1/4 inch thick.
- Remove the leaves off the stems of the basil and set them aside.

2. Assemble the Salad:

- Arrange the mozzarella and tomato slices in an alternating pattern on a serving plate.
- Evenly distribute the fresh basil leaves by tucking them between the tomato and mozzarella pieces.

3. Season and Dress:

- Pour extra virgin olive oil over the salad, being careful to coat the basil leaves, mozzarella, and tomatoes.

- You may optionally top the salad with a balsamic glaze to give it more sweetness and taste.
- Add a dash of salt and freshly ground black pepper to the salad.

4. Serve:

- Present the caprese salad right away as a bright and cheery starter or side dish.

Benefits:

- Low in Calories: Caprese salad is a light, calorie-conscious option that is both healthful and revitalizing.
- High in Antioxidants: Rich in phytonutrients and antioxidants that promote general health are tomatoes, basil, and extra-virgin olive oil.
- High-quality Protein: One good source of protein is fresh mozzarella.

Applications:

- Caprese salad works well as a side dish or as an appetizer before a bigger dinner.
- When coupled with a crusty baguette or toast, it may make a light and healthful lunch.
- Serve it as a vibrant and light accent to a summertime BBQ or picnic.

One-Pan Baked Salmon Recipe

Ingredients:

- 4 salmon fillets (6-8 ounces each), skin-on or skinless
- 1 pound baby potatoes, halved or quartered
- 1 bunch asparagus, woody ends trimmed
- 1 lemon, sliced into rounds
- 4 cloves garlic, minced
- 2 tablespoons olive oil
- 1 teaspoon dried oregano
- 1 teaspoon dried thyme
- Salt and freshly ground black pepper, to taste
- Fresh parsley, chopped, for garnish (optional)

Instructions:

1. Preheat the Oven:

- Preheat your oven to 400°F (200°C).

2. Prepare the Vegetables:

- Combine the baby potatoes cut in half, asparagus that has been trimmed, lemon slices, and chopped garlic in a big bowl.
- Add a drizzle of olive oil (1 tablespoon) to the veggies, and then salt, black pepper, dried thyme, and dried oregano. Toss to evenly coat the veggies.

3. Prep the Salmon:

- Transfer the salmon fillets to a platter and pour the last 1 tablespoon of olive oil over them. Add a little salt and black pepper to the fish.

4. Assemble the Dish:
- Arrange the seasoned veggies in an equal layer on a large baking sheet or ovenproof pan.
- Top the veggies with the salmon fillets. Put the salmon skin-side down if it has any.

5. Bake:
- After preheating the oven, place the baking sheet inside and bake for 15 to 20 minutes, or until the veggies are soft and have a light brown color and the salmon flakes easily with a fork.

6. Serve:
- Remove the one-pan cooked salmon from the oven with care, and if you'd like, garnish with freshly chopped parsley.

Benefits:
- High-quality Protein: Omega-3 fatty acids, which are good for the heart, and high-quality protein may both be found in salmon.
- Nutrient-Rich: The combined veggies in this meal provide a wealth of vitamins, minerals, and fiber.
- Convenience: Cooking and cleanup are made easier using the one-pan approach.

Applications:

- One-Pan Baked Salmon is a fantastic weekday dinner option for busy families or individuals looking for a healthy, quick meal.
- It's also a great dish to prepare when hosting guests, as it's impressive and minimal effort.
- Serve it alongside a simple salad or your favorite grain for a complete meal.

BLT Wrap Recipe

Ingredients:

For the BLT Filling:

- 4 large flour tortillas
- 8 slices of bacon, cooked until crispy
- 2 large tomatoes, sliced
- 2 cups fresh lettuce leaves (such as iceberg or Romaine), washed and patted dry
- Mayonnaise or your preferred spread
- Salt and black pepper, to taste

Instructions:

1. Cook the Bacon:

- Until it's crispy, cook the bacon in an oven or a pan, depending on your liking. After draining, place paper towels aside.

2. Prep the Ingredients:

- Cut the tomatoes into slender circles.
- Clean the lettuce and pat it dry.
- Arrange the flour tortillas in a neat line on a workspace.

3. Assemble the BLT Wraps:

- On each tortilla, spread a thin layer of mayonnaise or your preferred spread.
- Lay 2 slices of crispy bacon down the center of each tortilla.
- Add a generous layer of sliced tomatoes on top of the bacon.
- Place a handful of lettuce leaves over the tomatoes.

- Season with a pinch of salt and freshly ground black pepper if desired.

4. Roll the Wraps:

- To create a wrap, fold in the tortilla's sides and then tightly roll it up from the bottom.
- If necessary, use toothpicks to secure the wrap.

5. Serve:

- Immediately serve each BLT wrap by cutting it in half diagonally.

Benefits:

- Classic Flavor: The BLT wrap's flavor is pleasant and ageless since it mixes the traditional tastes of bacon, lettuce, and tomato with creamy mayonnaise.
- Protein and Fiber: Tomatoes and lettuce contribute fiber and vital nutrients, and bacon supplies protein.
- Customizable: You may use extras like cheese, avocado, or other spreads to add your own unique touch.

Applications:

- BLT wraps are perfect for a quick and satisfying lunch or dinner option.
- They are a popular choice for picnics, potlucks, and casual gatherings.
- These wraps can be enjoyed all year round, making them a versatile choice for any occasion.

Mushroom Risotto Recipe

Ingredients:

- 1 1/2 cups Arborio rice (or another short-grain rice suitable for risotto)
- 8 ounces (about 2 cups) fresh mushrooms (cremini, shiitake, or wild mushrooms), sliced
- 1 small onion, finely chopped
- 2 cloves garlic, minced
- 4 cups vegetable or chicken broth, warmed
- 1 cup dry white wine (optional)
- 2 tablespoons olive oil
- 2 tablespoons unsalted butter
- 1/2 cup grated Parmesan cheese
- Salt and black pepper, to taste
- Fresh parsley, chopped, for garnish (optional)

Instructions:

1. Sauté the Mushrooms:

- Heat the olive oil and 1 tablespoon of butter in a large skillet or wide saucepan over medium heat.
- Add the sliced mushrooms and sauté for 5 to 7 minutes, or until they lose their moisture and brown. Half of the cooked mushrooms should be removed and put aside.

2. Cook the Aromatics:

- In the same skillet, combine the chopped onion and minced garlic. Sauté for 2-3 minutes, or until the onion is translucent and fragrant.

3. Toast the Rice:

- Add the Arborio rice to the skillet and stir to coat it with the mushrooms, onions, and garlic. Cook for 1-2 minutes until the rice becomes slightly translucent at the edges.

4. Deglaze with Wine (optional):

- If using white wine, pour it into the skillet and stir until it's mostly absorbed by the rice.

5. Start Adding Broth:

- Begin adding the warm broth one ladleful at a time, stirring constantly. Wait until each addition of broth is mostly absorbed before adding more. Continue this process until the rice is creamy and tender. This will take about 18-20 minutes.

6. Finish the Risotto:

- Stir in the reserved sautéed mushrooms and the remaining 1 tablespoon of butter.
- Add the grated Parmesan cheese and stir until it's fully incorporated.
- Season with salt and black pepper to taste.

7. Garnish and Serve:

- Serve the mushroom risotto hot, garnished with chopped fresh parsley if desired.

Benefits:

- High in Vitamins and Fiber: A good supply of vitamins, antioxidants, and fiber is found in mushrooms.
- Creamy and Satisfying: Risotto's creamy texture and the umami taste of the mushrooms combine to create a comfort food classic.
- Adaptable: Risotto made from mushrooms may be eaten as a main entrée for vegetarians or as a side dish.

Applications:

- Mushroom risotto is an excellent side dish to complement various main courses like grilled chicken, steak, or seafood.
- It can also serve as a hearty, meatless main course, perfect for vegetarians and mushroom lovers.
- Mushroom risotto can be a delightful dish for special occasions and gatherings.

Spaghetti Aglio e Olio Recipe

Ingredients:

- 8 ounces (about 225g) spaghetti
- 4-5 cloves of garlic, thinly sliced
- 1/2 teaspoon red pepper flakes (adjust to taste)
- 1/3 cup extra-virgin olive oil
- 1/4 cup fresh Italian parsley, chopped
- Grated Pecorino Romano or Parmesan cheese, for garnish (optional)
- Salt and black pepper, to taste

Instructions:

1. Cook the Spaghetti:

- Bring a large pot of salted water to a boil.
- Add the spaghetti and cook according to the package instructions until it's al dente.
- Before draining, reserve about 1/2 cup of the pasta cooking water. Drain the spaghetti and set it aside.

2. Sauté the Garlic:

- In a large skillet, heat the olive oil over low heat.
- Add the thinly sliced garlic and red pepper flakes. Sauté gently, making sure not to let the garlic brown. This should take about 2-3 minutes.

3. Toss the Spaghetti:

- Add the cooked and drained spaghetti to the skillet with the garlic and red pepper flakes.

- Toss the spaghetti in the fragrant garlic and olive oil mixture. If it seems a little dry, add some of the reserved pasta cooking water to create a silky sauce.

4. Season and Garnish:

- Season the spaghetti with salt and black pepper to taste.
- Sprinkle the freshly chopped parsley over the top and toss the pasta again.

5. Serve:

- Divide the Spaghetti Aglio e Olio onto plates and, if desired, garnish with grated Pecorino Romano or Parmesan cheese.

Benefits:

- **Quick and Simple:** Spaghetti Aglio e Olio is a quick and easy pasta dish, perfect for busy weeknights.
- **Heart-Healthy:** Olive oil is a source of heart-healthy monounsaturated fats, while garlic offers potential health benefits.
- **Versatile:** You can enjoy it as a straightforward pasta dish or add ingredients like shrimp, cherry tomatoes, or spinach for variety.

Applications:

- Spaghetti Aglio e Olio is perfect as a simple, satisfying meal on its own, especially when you're short on time.
- It can serve as a base for a variety of add-ins, such as grilled chicken, shrimp, or

other proteins, making it a versatile and customizable dish.

- Ideal for a light lunch or dinner with a fresh salad or garlic bread on the side.

Quick Veggie Fried Rice Recipe

Ingredients:

- 2 cups cooked and cooled white or brown rice (preferably a day old)
- 2 tablespoons vegetable oil
- 1 cup mixed vegetables (e.g., diced carrots, peas, corn, and bell peppers)
- 2 cloves garlic, minced
- 1/2 cup diced onion
- 2-3 tablespoons soy sauce (adjust to taste)
- 1 teaspoon sesame oil
- 2 eggs, beaten
- Salt and black pepper, to taste
- Sliced green onions or chopped cilantro, for garnish (optional)

Instructions:

1. Prepare the Rice:

- If you don't have day-old rice, cook the rice according to package instructions and allow it to cool in the refrigerator for at least an hour before using. Cold rice works best for fried rice.

2. Sauté the Vegetables:

- Heat 1 tablespoon of vegetable oil in a large skillet or wok over medium-high heat.

- Add the diced onion and mixed vegetables to the skillet. Stir-fry for about 3-4 minutes until the vegetables are tender.
- Add the minced garlic and cook for an additional 30 seconds until fragrant.

3. Add the Rice:

- Add the cooked and cooled rice to the skillet with the sautéed vegetables.
- Use a spatula to break up any clumps of rice and stir everything together.

4. Season with Soy Sauce and Sesame Oil:

- Drizzle the soy sauce and sesame oil over the rice and vegetables. Stir to evenly coat and flavor the dish.

5. Scramble the Eggs:

- Push the rice and vegetable mixture to one side of the skillet and add the remaining 1 tablespoon of vegetable oil to the empty side.
- Pour the beaten eggs into the oil and quickly scramble them until they're fully cooked.

6. Combine and Season:

- Stir the scrambled eggs into the rice and vegetable mixture.
- Season with salt and black pepper to taste.

7. Garnish and Serve:

- Remove the skillet from heat and garnish the Quick Veggie Fried Rice with sliced green onions or chopped cilantro if desired.

Benefits:

- Quick and Easy: This dish makes a delicious dinner that can be prepared quickly on a weekday.
- Versatile: Feel free to alter the flavors and veggies to your taste.
- Balanced: The combination of vegetables, protein, and carbs in Quick Veggie Fried Rice makes it a good choice.

Applications:

- You may serve Quick Veggie Fried Rice as a side dish to go well with grilled chicken, shrimp, or tofu.
- It makes a great solo dish for a light and filling supper.
- It's a fantastic way to finish off leftover rice and veggies from other dinners.

Turkey and Avocado Sandwich Recipe

Ingredients:

- 2 slices of whole-grain bread or your choice of bread
- 4-6 slices of lean turkey breast
- 1/2 ripe avocado, sliced
- 2-3 lettuce leaves (such as romaine or butter lettuce)
- 2-3 slices of tomato
- 2-3 slices of red onion (optional)
- Mustard, mayonnaise, or your preferred spread
- Salt and black pepper, to taste

Instructions:

1. Prepare the Ingredients:

- Wash and dry the lettuce leaves.
- Slice the avocado, tomato, and red onion (if using).
- Lay out two slices of bread on a clean surface.

2. Build the Sandwich:

- On one slice of bread, spread a thin layer of mustard, mayonnaise, or your preferred spread.
- Layer the turkey slices on top of the spread.
- Add the avocado slices, followed by the tomato slices.

- Place the lettuce leaves on top of the tomato.
- If desired, add the slices of red onion for an extra kick.
- Season with a pinch of salt and freshly ground black pepper.

3. Assemble the Sandwich:

- Place the second slice of bread on top of the sandwich ingredients to form a complete sandwich.

4. Cut and Serve:

- Use a sharp knife to cut the sandwich in half diagonally or into smaller portions.
- Serve your Turkey and Avocado Sandwich immediately.

Benefits:

- Protein: Turkey that is lean is a good source of protein.
- Good Fats: Avocados are high in nutrients and provide good monounsaturated fats.
- Fiber and Nutrients: Vital fiber, vitamins, and minerals are provided by whole-grain bread and veggies.

Applications:

- A turkey and avocado sandwich is a great alternative for a filling and fast lunch or dinner.
- It makes a tasty and portable meal for hikes, picnics, and packed lunches.
- Add cheese, bacon, or your preferred spreads and condiments to personalize it.

Easy Egg Fried Rice Recipe

Ingredients:

- 2 cups cooked and cooled white rice (preferably a day old)
- 2 large eggs
- 2 tablespoons vegetable oil
- 1/2 cup mixed vegetables (e.g., peas, carrots, corn)
- 2 cloves garlic, minced
- 2-3 tablespoons soy sauce (adjust to taste)
- Salt and black pepper, to taste
- Sliced green onions for garnish (optional)

Instructions:

1. Prepare the Rice:

- If you don't have day-old rice, cook the rice according to package instructions and allow it to cool in the refrigerator for at least an hour before using. Cold rice works best for fried rice.

2. Sauté the Vegetables:

- In a large skillet or wok, heat 1 tablespoon of vegetable oil over medium-high heat.
- Add the mixed vegetables and minced garlic to the skillet. Stir-fry for about 3-4 minutes until the vegetables are tender.

3. Scramble the Eggs:

- Push the sautéed vegetables to one side of the skillet and add the remaining 1

tablespoon of vegetable oil to the empty side.
- Crack the eggs into the oil and quickly scramble them until they're mostly cooked but still slightly runny.

4. Combine with Rice:
- Add the cooked and cooled rice to the skillet with the scrambled eggs and sautéed vegetables. Stir to combine all the ingredients.

5. Season with Soy Sauce:
- Drizzle the soy sauce over the rice and continue to stir-fry until everything is well mixed and the rice is heated through.

6. Season and Garnish:
- Season the fried rice with salt and black pepper to taste.
- If desired, garnish with sliced green onions for a fresh, oniony flavor and visual appeal.

7. Serve:
- Serve your Easy Egg Fried Rice hot as a side dish or add cooked chicken, shrimp, or tofu for a complete meal.

Benefits:
- Quick and Easy: This dish makes a delicious dinner that can be prepared quickly on a weekday.
- Versatile: You may alter the flavors, meats, and veggies to your preference.

- Balanced: A combination of vegetables, protein, and carbs may be found in Easy Egg Fried Rice.

Applications:

- Simple Egg Fried Rice is an excellent side dish on its own or as a foundation for your preferred protein, such shrimp, chicken, or tofu.
- If you're pressed for time, it can be served as a fast lunch or dinner.
- It's a fantastic way to use up leftover vegetables and grains.

Crispy Chicken Tenders Recipe

Ingredients:

For the Chicken Tenders:

- 1 pound boneless, skinless chicken breast or tenders
- 1 cup all-purpose flour
- 2 large eggs
- 1 cup breadcrumbs (seasoned or plain)
- 1 teaspoon paprika
- 1/2 teaspoon garlic powder
- 1/2 teaspoon onion powder
- Salt and black pepper, to taste
- Vegetable oil, for frying

For Dipping Sauce (Optional):

- Ketchup, honey mustard, BBQ sauce, or your preferred dipping sauce

Instructions:

1. Prep the Chicken:

- Cut the chicken breast into strips to make chicken tenders. If you're using pre-cut tenders, you can skip this step.

2. Set Up a Breading Station:

- In three (3) separate shallow dishes, place the following:
    - Dish 1: All-purpose flour seasoned with salt and black pepper.
    - Dish 2: Beaten eggs.

- Dish 3: Breadcrumbs mixed with paprika, garlic powder, onion powder, salt, and black pepper.

3. Bread the Chicken:

- Take a chicken tender and coat it in the flour, shaking off any excess.
- Dip it into the beaten eggs, ensuring it's fully coated.
- Transfer it to the breadcrumb mixture, pressing the breadcrumbs onto the chicken to adhere.

4. Heat the Oil:

- In a large skillet or frying pan, heat about 1/2 inch of vegetable oil over medium-high heat until it reaches 350-375°F (175-190°C).

5. Fry the Chicken Tenders:

- Carefully place the breaded chicken tenders into the hot oil, a few at a time, making sure not to overcrowd the pan.
- Fry for about 3-4 minutes per side, or until the chicken is golden brown and cooked through with an internal temperature of 165°F (74°C).

6. Drain and Serve:

- Remove the crispy chicken tenders from the oil and place them on a plate lined with paper towels to drain any excess oil.
- Serve the chicken tenders hot with your favorite dipping sauce.

Benefits:

- Crispy and Delectable: Crispy Chicken Tenders are a crowd favorite because of their crispy outside and juicy, tender within.
- Rich in Protein: This meal is a filling and healthy option because chicken is a lean source of protein.
- Kid-Friendly: This meal is a great choice for the whole family because it appeals to both adults and children.

Applications:

- Crispy Chicken Tenders are a favorite for kid-friendly dinners, get-togethers, and game day snacks.
- They may be served as a main course with fries, coleslaw, or a salad.
- They also go well with salads, sandwiches, and wraps.

Mushroom and Spinach Omelette Recipe

Ingredients:

- 3 large eggs
- 1/2 cup sliced mushrooms (e.g., cremini, button, or shiitake)
- 1 cup fresh spinach leaves, washed and roughly chopped
- 1/4 cup diced onion
- 1/4 cup shredded cheese (e.g., cheddar, Swiss, or feta)
- 2 tablespoons butter or cooking oil
- Salt and black pepper, to taste
- Fresh herbs, such as chives or parsley, for garnish (optional)

Instructions:

1. Prepare the Fillings:

- In a small skillet, heat 1 tablespoon of butter or cooking oil over medium heat.
- Add the diced onion and sliced mushrooms. Sauté for about 3-4 minutes, or until the mushrooms are tender and the onions are translucent.
- Add the chopped spinach to the skillet and cook for an additional 1-2 minutes, or until wilted. Season with salt and black pepper. Set the cooked vegetables aside.

2. Whisk the Eggs:

- Crack the eggs into a bowl and whisk them until the yolks and whites are fully combined. Season with a pinch of salt and black pepper.

3. Cook the Omelette:

- In a separate skillet, melt the remaining 1 tablespoon of butter or heat the cooking oil over medium-high heat.
- Pour the whisked eggs into the skillet, ensuring they spread out evenly.

4. Add the Fillings:

- As the edges of the omelette start to set, spoon the cooked mushroom, spinach, and onion mixture onto one-half of the omelette.
- Sprinkle the shredded cheese over the filling.

5. Fold and Serve:

- When the omelette is mostly set but still slightly runny on top, carefully fold it in half using a spatula.
- Cook for an additional minute, or until the cheese is melted, and the omelette is fully set.

6. Garnish and Serve:

- Slide the Mushroom and Spinach Omelette onto a plate.
- Garnish with fresh herbs, such as chives or parsley, if desired.

Benefits:

- Protein and Veggies: The minerals and fiber from spinach and mushrooms are combined with the protein from eggs in this omelette.

- Quick and Nutritious: Omelettes are a fast, adaptable, and wholesome alternative for brunch or breakfast.
- Low in Carbs: Omelettes are a good fit for low-carb or keto diets since they naturally contain little carbs.

Applications:

- Mushroom and Spinach Omelette is perfect for breakfast or brunch.
- It can be served with toast, a side salad, or a breakfast potato dish.
- Customize it with additional ingredients like bell peppers, tomatoes, or different types of cheese.

Baked Ziti Recipe

Ingredients:

For the Ziti and Sauce:

- 12 ounces (about 3 cups) ziti or penne pasta
- 1 tablespoon olive oil
- 1 pound ground beef or Italian sausage (optional)
- 1 small onion, chopped
- 3 cloves garlic, minced
- 24 ounces (about 3 cups) marinara sauce
- 1 teaspoon dried oregano
- 1 teaspoon dried basil
- Salt and black pepper, to taste

For the Cheese Mixture:

- 15 ounces (about 2 cups) ricotta cheese
- 1 egg
- 1/4 cup grated Parmesan cheese
- 2 cups shredded mozzarella cheese

Instructions:

1. Cook the Pasta:

- Preheat your oven to 375°F (190°C).
- Cook the ziti or penne pasta according to the package instructions until it's al dente. Drain and set aside.

2. Prepare the Meat Sauce (Optional):

- In a large skillet, heat the olive oil over medium heat.

- If you're using ground beef or Italian sausage, add it to the skillet and cook until browned. Remove any excess fat.
- Add the chopped onion and minced garlic to the skillet, and sauté until the onion is translucent.
- Stir in the marinara sauce, dried oregano, and dried basil. Season with salt and black pepper to taste. Simmer for about 10 minutes.

3. Make the Cheese Mixture:

- In a separate bowl, combine the ricotta cheese, egg, and grated Parmesan cheese.

4. Assemble the Baked Ziti:

- In a large baking dish, spread a thin layer of the meat sauce or marinara sauce (if using).
- Add half of the cooked ziti or penne pasta to the dish.
- Spoon half of the cheese mixture over the pasta and spread it evenly.
- Sprinkle half of the shredded mozzarella cheese over the cheese mixture.
- Repeat the layers with the remaining pasta, cheese mixture, and mozzarella cheese.

5. Bake:

- Cover the baking dish with aluminum foil and bake in the preheated oven for about 25 minutes.

- Remove the foil and bake for an additional 10-15 minutes or until the cheese is melted and bubbly, and the dish is heated through.

6. Serve:

- Let the Baked Ziti rest for a few minutes before serving.

Benefits:

- Make-Ahead: Made ahead of time, baked ziti is a terrific meal prep option that delivers both calcium and protein from the cheese and the meat.
- It is a hearty and warming pasta dish that is excellent for fulfilling your appetites.

Applications:

- A side salad or garlic bread go well with baked ziti, which makes a filling main course.
- It's a great option for informal get-togethers, family get-togethers, and potlucks.
- Baked ziti leftovers make a great lunch or supper when warmed.

Grilled Cheese and Tomato Soup Recipe

Ingredients:

For the Grilled Cheese:

- 4 slices of your preferred bread (white, whole wheat, sourdough, or multigrain)
- 4 slices of cheese (cheddar, American, Swiss, or your favorite type)
- 2 tablespoons butter, softened

For the Tomato Soup:

- 1 tablespoon olive oil
- 1 small onion, chopped
- 2 cloves garlic, minced
- 1 can (28 ounces) crushed tomatoes
- 2 cups vegetable or chicken broth
- 1 teaspoon dried basil
- 1 teaspoon dried oregano
- Salt and black pepper, to taste
- 1/4 cup heavy cream (optional)
- Fresh basil leaves, for garnish (optional)

Instructions:

1. Prepare the Tomato Soup:

- In a large pot, heat the olive oil over medium heat.
- Add the chopped onion and sauté for 3-4 minutes, or until the onion is translucent.
- Stir in the minced garlic and sauté for an additional 30 seconds, until fragrant.

- Add the crushed tomatoes, vegetable or chicken broth, dried basil, dried oregano, salt, and black pepper. Stir to combine.
- Bring the soup to a simmer and let it cook for about 10-15 minutes, allowing the flavors to meld. If desired, stir in the heavy cream for a creamier soup.

2. Make the Grilled Cheese:

- Lay out the four slices of bread.
- Place a slice of cheese between two slices of bread to form two sandwiches.
- Butter the outer sides of each sandwich.

3. Grill the Sandwiches:

- In a skillet or on a griddle over medium heat, place the sandwiches, buttered side down.
- Grill for 3-4 minutes on each side, or until the bread is golden brown, and the cheese inside is melted.

4. Serve:

- Serve the Grilled Cheese alongside the Tomato Soup, garnished with fresh basil leaves if desired.

Benefits:

- Comfort Food: A traditional comfort food combo that appeals to both adults and children alike is grilled cheese and tomato soup.
- High in Lycopene: Lycopene is an antioxidant linked to a number of health

advantages, and tomato soup is a strong source of this nutrient.

- Protein and Calcium: The grilled cheese sandwich's cheese offers both of these nutrients.

Applications:

- Grilled cheese and tomato soup is a delicious choice for lunch or dinner during the cooler months.
- It may be eaten as a quick and satisfying meal at home or packed as a lunch for work or school.
- This classic combo is a hit at cafés and restaurants and is a great option for parties or get-togethers.

Honey Garlic Shrimp Recipe

Ingredients:

For the Honey Garlic Shrimp:

- 1 pound large shrimp, peeled and deveined
- 2 tablespoons honey
- 3 cloves garlic, minced
- 2 tablespoons soy sauce
- 1 tablespoon rice vinegar
- 1/2 teaspoon ginger, minced (optional)
- 2 tablespoons olive oil or cooking oil
- Salt and black pepper, to taste
- Red pepper flakes (optional, for heat)
- Fresh parsley or green onions, for garnish (optional)

Instructions:

1. Prepare the Shrimp:

- Pat the shrimp dry with paper towels.
- Season the shrimp with salt and black pepper to taste.

2. Make the Honey Garlic Sauce:

- In a small bowl, whisk together the honey, minced garlic, soy sauce, rice vinegar, and ginger (if using). Add red pepper flakes if you prefer a spicy kick.

3. Sauté the Shrimp:

- Heat the olive oil or cooking oil in a large skillet or wok over medium-high heat.

- Add the seasoned shrimp to the hot skillet and cook for 1-2 minutes on each side until they turn pink and opaque.
- Remove the cooked shrimp from the skillet and set them aside.

4. Create the Sauce:

- In the same skillet, add the honey garlic sauce mixture.
- Cook the sauce for about 2-3 minutes, or until it thickens slightly and becomes glossy.

5. Combine Shrimp and Sauce:

- Return the cooked shrimp to the skillet and toss them in the honey garlic sauce to coat evenly.

6. Serve:

- Serve the Honey Garlic Shrimp immediately, garnished with fresh parsley or green onions if desired.

Benefits:

- Protein: Shrimp is a high-quality, low-calorie source of protein.
- Flavorful: The ideal balance of savory and sweet tastes is provided by honey garlic sauce.
- Fast and Simple: This recipe comes together quickly, making it an excellent choice for a midweek supper.

Applications:

- Quinoa or steamed rice can be served alongside Honey Garlic Shrimp as a main course.
- It's a delicious choice for a simple and quick supper. It can also be served as an appetizer at events like parties.

Mediterranean Hummus Wrap Recipe

Ingredients:

For the Wrap:

- 1 large whole-grain or spinach tortilla (or your preferred type)
- 1/4 cup hummus
- 1/2 cup mixed salad greens (e.g., baby spinach, arugula, or mixed greens)
- 1/4 cup cucumber, thinly sliced
- 1/4 cup cherry tomatoes, halved
- 1/4 cup red bell pepper, thinly sliced
- 1/4 cup red onion, thinly sliced
- 2-3 tablespoons Kalamata olives, pitted and sliced (optional)
- 2-3 tablespoons crumbled feta cheese (optional)
- Fresh parsley or cilantro leaves, for garnish (optional)
- Olive oil and balsamic vinegar, for drizzling (optional)
- Salt and black pepper, to taste

Instructions:

1. Prepare the Ingredients:

- Lay the tortilla flat on a clean surface.
- Spread a layer of hummus over the entire surface of the tortilla.
- In the center of the tortilla, place the mixed salad greens, cucumber slices, cherry tomatoes, red bell pepper, red

onion, Kalamata olives (if using), and crumbled feta cheese (if using).

- Drizzle with olive oil and balsamic vinegar if desired.
- Season with salt and black pepper to taste.
- Garnish with fresh parsley or cilantro leaves if desired.

2. Fold and Roll the Wrap:

- Carefully fold in the sides of the tortilla.
- Starting from the bottom, tightly roll up the tortilla, enclosing the fillings.

3. Cut and Serve:

- Using a sharp knife, cut the Mediterranean Hummus Wrap in half diagonally or into smaller portions.
- Serve immediately, or wrap in parchment paper or foil for a convenient, portable meal.

Benefits:

- Nutrient-Rich: This wrap is loaded with fiber and nutritious components, including veggies.
- Plant-Based Protein: One good source of plant-based protein is hummus.
- Versatile: You may alter the contents to fit your tastes, so it can accommodate a range of dietary requirements.

Applications:

- The Mediterranean Hummus Wrap is a convenient and filling meal that can be

eaten at work, school, or on the road. It's perfect for a quick and healthful lunch or supper.
- It may be brought to potlucks, picnics, or dinners with a Mediterranean theme.

Asian Noodle Salad Recipe

Ingredients:

For the Salad:

- 8 ounces (about 225g) of your choice of noodles (e.g., spaghetti, soba, rice noodles)
- 2 cups mixed fresh vegetables (e.g., bell peppers, cucumber, carrots, snap peas, or edamame)
- 1/4 cup fresh cilantro leaves, chopped
- 1/4 cup fresh mint leaves, chopped
- 2-3 green onions, thinly sliced
- 1/4 cup chopped peanuts or cashews (optional)
- Sesame seeds, for garnish (optional)

For the Dressing:

- 3 tablespoons soy sauce
- 2 tablespoons rice vinegar
- 2 tablespoons sesame oil
- 1-2 tablespoons honey or maple syrup (adjust to taste)
- 1-2 cloves garlic, minced
- 1 teaspoon fresh ginger, minced
- Red pepper flakes or Sriracha, to taste (optional)
- Salt and black pepper, to taste

Instructions:

1. Cook the Noodles:

- Cook the noodles according to the package instructions. Drain and rinse them under cold water to stop the cooking process. Set aside.

2. Prepare the Vegetables:

- Wash and chop the fresh vegetables into thin strips or bite-sized pieces.

3. Make the Dressing:

- In a small bowl, whisk together the soy sauce, rice vinegar, sesame oil, honey or maple syrup, minced garlic, minced ginger, red pepper flakes or Sriracha (if using), salt, and black pepper. Adjust the sweetness and spiciness to your liking.

4. Assemble the Salad:

- In a large bowl, combine the cooked and cooled noodles, chopped vegetables, cilantro, mint, and green onions.
- Pour the dressing over the salad and toss everything together until well coated.
- If desired, add the chopped peanuts or cashews for crunch.

5. Garnish and Serve:

- Garnish the Asian Noodle Salad with sesame seeds and serve immediately.

Benefits:

- Versatile: You may alter the ingredients to suit your taste and dietary requirements.
- Light and Fresh: Asian Noodle Salad is a light and delicious dish full of fresh veggies and herbs.
- Balanced: This salad offers a decent ratio of carbs, fiber, and minerals.

Applications:

- Asian Noodle Salad is a great side dish to bring to potlucks, picnics, and barbecues.
- It's a terrific option for a filling and light lunch or dinner on its own.
- To make it a full dinner, you can add grilled chicken, shrimp, tofu, or other proteins.

Quick Beef Tacos Recipe

Ingredients:

For the Beef Filling:

- 1 pound ground beef
- 1 small onion, finely chopped
- 2 cloves garlic, minced
- 1 packet taco seasoning mix or use your own blend (chili powder, cumin, paprika, oregano, salt, and pepper)
- 1/4 cup water

For Assembling Tacos:

- 8 small taco shells or soft tortillas
- 1 cup shredded lettuce
- 1 cup diced tomatoes
- 1/2 cup shredded cheddar cheese
- 1/2 cup sour cream
- 1/4 cup chopped fresh cilantro (optional)
- Salsa, guacamole, or hot sauce (optional)
- Lime wedges (optional)

Instructions:

1. Cook the Beef Filling:

- Add the ground beef to a large pan over medium-high heat, and cook until it begins to brown.
- After the beef is thoroughly browned and the onions are transparent, add the finely chopped onion and minced garlic to the meat.
- Pour out any remaining grease in the skillet.

- Add the water and stir in the taco seasoning mix or make your own mixture. Simmer for a few minutes to allow the flavors to mingle and the mixture to thicken. If necessary, adjust the seasoning.

2. Assemble the Tacos:

- Warm the taco shells or tortillas in the oven or microwave according to the package instructions.
- In each shell, add a portion of the cooked beef filling.
- Top the beef with shredded lettuce, diced tomatoes, shredded cheddar cheese, and any optional toppings you prefer, such as sour cream, cilantro, salsa, guacamole, or hot sauce.

3. Serve:

- Serve your Quick Beef Tacos with lime wedges for a fresh squeeze of citrus if desired.

Benefits:

- Fast and Easy: These Quick Beef Tacos are a great option for hectic weekday dinners since they can be prepared quickly.
- Adaptable: You may change the toppings to fit your tastes, so it can accommodate a variety of dietary requirements.
- High in Protein: Beef is a rich source of protein.

Applications:

- Quick Beef Tacos provide a flexible and filling lunch or supper on their own.
- They're also a great option for parties, get-togethers, and game day snacks.
- You might set up a taco bar with different toppings, allowing visitors to put up their own tacos.

CONCLUSION

As we wrap up the "Essential Fast Feast Repeat Cookbook," we take a moment to appreciate the incredible experience that we have all shared. We've taken you on an investigation of tastes, efficiency, and health-conscious eating via the pages of this cookbook.

It has been our honor to lead you down a path where quick, tasty, and low-calorie meals come together to create a way of life that embraces taste and wellbeing.

We are aware that losing weight is sometimes a difficult journey, but it is also one full of successes and little wins. You've learned that eating in a way that is healthful doesn't have to mean sacrificing taste. It may be a joyful feast of tastes and sensual pleasures that satiate the body and the spirit.

Through "Essential Fast Feast Repeat," you've discovered the keys to a well-rounded, long-lasting, and pleasurable weight loss strategy. You now know that eating well can be quick and fulfilling.
You now understand that making steady, educated decisions rather than taking extreme actions is the key to improving your health.

We really hope that the guides and recipes you've found here will remain your reliable allies as you work to lead a better lifestyle. To help you incorporate these practices into your everyday life, we invite you to fast, feast, and repeat these rituals.

May every meal serve as a milestone in your pursuit of well-being, and may you relish the tastes as well as the advancements you make along the path.

We thus urge you to keep discovering the fascinating realm of healthy food and weight-friendly living as you put this cookbook away. It's important to keep in mind that you are responsible for your own health and wellbeing, and the "Essential Fast Feast Repeat Cookbook" is here to help you along the journey.

We encourage you to use the knowledge you've learned about cooking here and customize it to suit your own preferences and requirements. Your daily and meal-by-meal decisions set the course for long-lasting transformation.

We are ecstatic to have shared in your journey, and we eagerly anticipate the many more experiences you will have as you work toward being a better, happier version of yourself.

We appreciate your participation in the "Essential Fast Feast Repeat Cookbook" event. Good luck on your journey to becoming a better, happier version of yourself, and until we cross paths over dinner, good appétit.